MY 6 SIMPLE SECRETS TO SHED FAT FAST!

LEGAL DISCLAIMER

COPYRIGHT

TABLE OF CONTENTS

ACKNOWLEDGMENTS

I WANT TO THANK GOD FOR THE ABILITY AND THE KNOWLEDGE THAT I HAVE BEEN GIVEN THE GIFT OF CREATING THIS BOOK. I THANK MY SUPPORT SYSTEM FOR HELPING ME THROUGH THE PROCESS. I THANK MY FAMILY FOR LOVING ME DESPITE MY FLAWS. I ALSO THANK YOU, THE READER, FOR TAKING THE TIME OUT OF YOUR BUSY LIFE TO READ THIS BOOK.

I AM NOT A DOCTOR AND MY WORDS ARE PURELY FROM EXPERIENCE.

INTRODUCTION

The number one thing that people assume when you are overweight is that you've somehow eaten a pig and they can't figure out how. Honestly, I am so sick and tired of this perception of being "fat" and it's no longer funny when someone makes jokes about your eating habits or the way you fit into your clothes.

About 5 years ago, I was an overweight, unhappy loser and yes, I say a loser because at the time, I was not genuinely ready to win over my body. I was allowing those negative perpetual thoughts to stump me right into bad shape. At 317 pounds, you'd think a person would be ready for a change, but nope. That wasn't me. For as long as I can remember I enjoyed my pity party and used it as an excuse to stay fat and unhealthy.

So, by now you are wondering, what's changed? Why should you listen to me rant or continue to read this book? What good will it for you? Well, if someone had introduced a book like this to me some odd years ago, I would have had similar thoughts floating into my mind.

The truth is, we are all winners deep within. The problem is… the fatter you are, the further you are from that inner self.

I have created this book as a way for you to challenge yourself to step outside of your comfort zone. Even if for only 6 minutes a day, you follow along with each step of this book, you WILL live a better life.

You see, it's thanks to these very steps that I have managed to shed over 100 pounds and have maintained keeping it off!

Truth be told, I've invested in so many products that over promised what they would help me to do and under sold, I've also damn near starved myself to death by counting my calories. Of all these things, there seems to be only 1 solution and that is listening to my own body.

I know, you're probably thinking that your body is the one telling you to eat all of that bull-crap that is keeping you where you are right now. STOP now! Quit lying to yourself. Do you have a desire to be fat deep within or thin? So, if you have a desire to be thin, healthy and fit… don't you think that your inner self would be leading you toward it?

It's time my friend! Time for you to quit making excuses for why you are not putting yourself first and make the decision to live a more happy, healthy and fulfilling life.

If you are ready to begin this journey and take your life a little more serious, turn the page and let's begin.

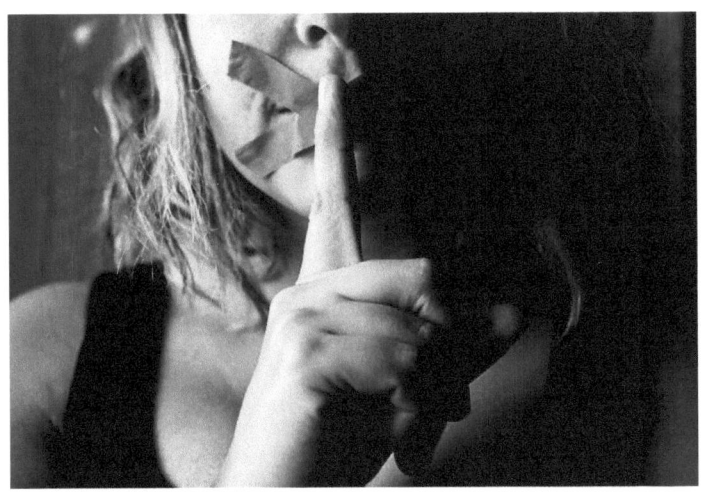

STEP 1
SILENCE... IT'S GOLDEN

When was the last time you sat back and enjoyed the nature of Silence itself?

Taking the necessary time that you need in order to reflect allows for better alignment with your inner peace. Too often, I hear people say, "I don't have time to sit still." It is this belief that causes you pure inner chaos and then, next thing you know your off on a tangent somewhere, forgetting what you were doing in the first place.

Did you know, that you do not control your thoughts? Have you ever told someone, "Let me think about it?" Well, what you are really doing is allowing the thought to settle as you distinguish whether or not that idea is in alignment with your values.

The average person has about 60,000 thoughts per day. Those thoughts are on autopilot. The only way to determine whether the ideas that are passing resonate with your inner self is to be aware of how you feel. When you are aware of how you feel, then you can make a decision based on your inner compass.

By adding Silence to your day, you can be sure to become more aware and more conscious of how you feel.

MEDITATION

Each morning, I begin with a 15-minute body scan meditation. This allows me to awaken my mind and allow the alignment between my mind and body to take place. Slowly and one by one, I gather my senses into each part of my body.

Quickly, I become more aware of the lightness in my body. This, my friend, is your natural state of being.

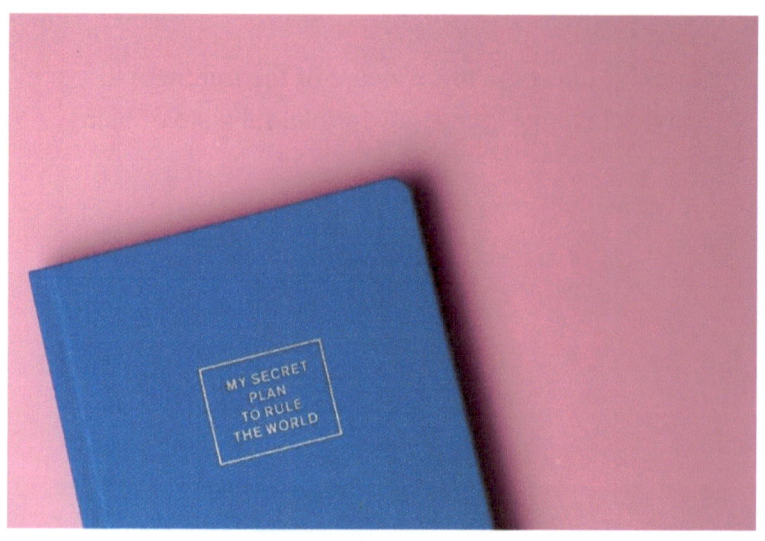

STEP 2
AFFIRM IT!

There is Power in every word you speak and every word you speak is an affirmation. An affirmation is a statement that declares something as true.

What are you declaring as true in your life? Do you say things like, "I am tired," "I am broke" or "I am fat?" Are these ideas ones that you want to be true for you? What thoughts about 'You' ponder your mind? What do you tell yourself about the way you are right now? Are you your own best friend or your worst enemy?

Believe it or not, your words have everything to do with where you stand right now. I say this because your words are evidence of what your inner chatter is.

J.O.U.R.N.A.L.

Every day, I journal these affirmations of mine out in a notebook that I find most attractive.

Writing affirmations out on paper allows you to see what you say about yourself and this will give you a good idea of what you'd rather be saying about yourself.

What are your goals? How long do you think it will take for you to reach these goals and says who? Who is your ideal self and what would you say to you right now? These are the things that you should journal.

You can also access FREE Journal Prompts at http://mysacredpleasures.com/journal-writing-prompts/.

Judgment Free Stop over criticizing yourself and everything you say and do. Why do you keep judging yourself because you are not where you think you should be right now? Where is that exactly? Without judgment, keep track of your thoughts on paper and be sure to reflect on them regularly.

Observation What you believe leads to what you think about and what you think about leads to how you feel. If you can be aware of how you are feeling, then you can determine which ideas are causing you to feel what. Keep track of these observations in your journal.

Understanding Avoid making your journal just a way to vent out your negative emotions. Be sure that as you dish out the negative, that you analyze those thoughts and come to a place of understanding within yourself, therefore manifesting as inner peace.

"Treat you as you are your own best friend. Don't beat yourself up."

Revelation This process can often lead to us having revelations about your dreams, your goals and your aspirations. Journaling can help you get in touch with your core self.

Needs Assessment Keeping a daily journal makes it easier to notice problems and potential solutions, as the simple act of writing something down can make it seem simpler and clearer. Keeping everything bottled up can be extremely harmful, and just putting pen to paper can sometimes be all that is needed to release some pressure.

Awareness Writing down your experiences helps you to take a wider perspective on your life, as well as reminding you of problem areas and things you must be grateful for. Raising awareness of these areas is the first step towards making the necessary changes and appreciating what you have.

Life Quality Journaling is known to be an effective way to destress and decrease anxiety. Just a few minutes a day can have a major impact on health and happiness.

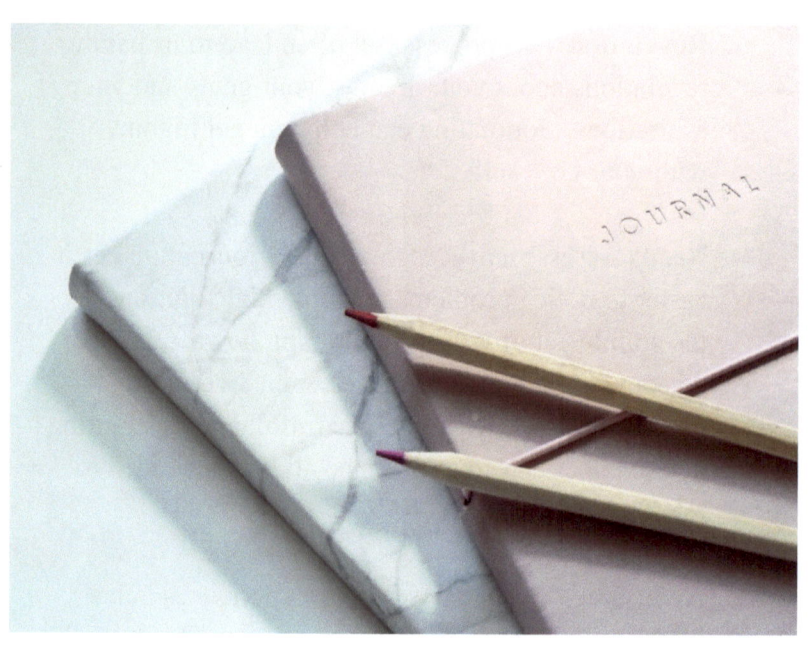

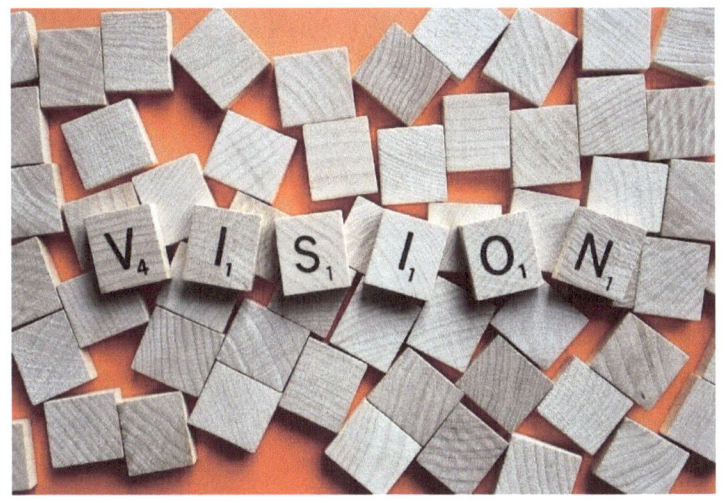

STEP 3
YOUR VISION

I'm sure you have at some point in your life you've created a vision board or thought about creating one. Well, my friend, now is the time to get it all out into a picture.

Visualize your life and create it, literally.

Do you truly understand the power of your mind? After 17 seconds of pondering or focusing on a particular thought, that idea takes on a momentum of its own and is followed up by another similar idea. Do that for about 60 seconds and you will begin to see evidence of this idea manifest in your body and in your life.

The feelings from these thoughts begin to take over us and we can begin to convince ourselves in the "reality" of that idea.

FAKE IT 'TILL YOU MAKE IT

If you have ever heard that term, fake it 'till you make it, then you will totally resonate with what I am about to tell you…

When you focus on a subject long enough, you will begin to see evidence of it all around you in your physical world. What we appear to be doing is bringing the subject at hand to the forefront of our mind and pretending as if it is apart of our Now experience. On a subconscious level, that message is received and the body begins to feel the excitement behind our revelation.

That, my friend, is creation at its most powerful!

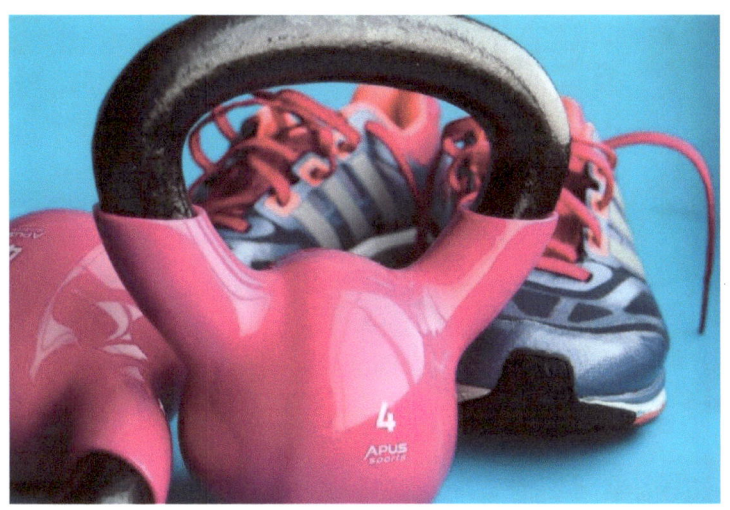

STEP 4
EXERCISE

Even if it's only for 7 minutes per day, you should have some sort of physical activity in your routine. You may not know the power of just 7 minutes per day, but listen, I started out at 317lbs with 4 minutes per day and here I stand, 100lbs lighter.

If I can do it, you can too!

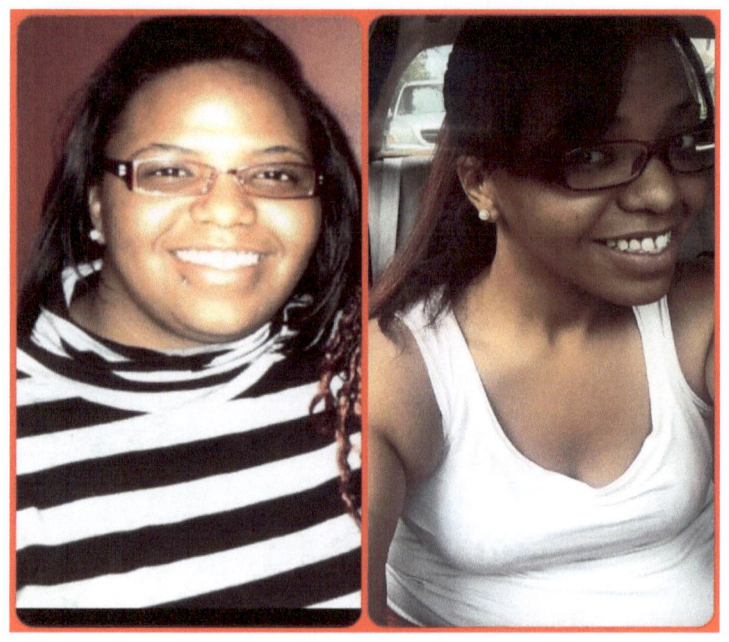

PICK WHAT FITS

When I first began my journey, I started with 4-minute cardio workouts and yoga for weight-loss. Now days, I love a good yoga for flexibility routines and some Pilates. There are some great dance workouts on YouTube that will help you to burn some calories while gettin' yo' groove on. I like to switch and mix it up, so my advise to you is to find what works for you and stick with it, but every now and then switch it up.

You can also check out my online one on one workout sessions, packed with high energy, high intensity workout routines created for you and me to do together. Book your spot at http://mysacredpleasures.com/services/.

DRINK PLENTY WATER

Make sure you are getting plenty of water in a day. You should be drinking half of your body weight in fluid ounces.

For help calculating, taking your weight, divide by 2 and the result is how much water you should intake. The average bottle of water holds 16 fluid ounces.

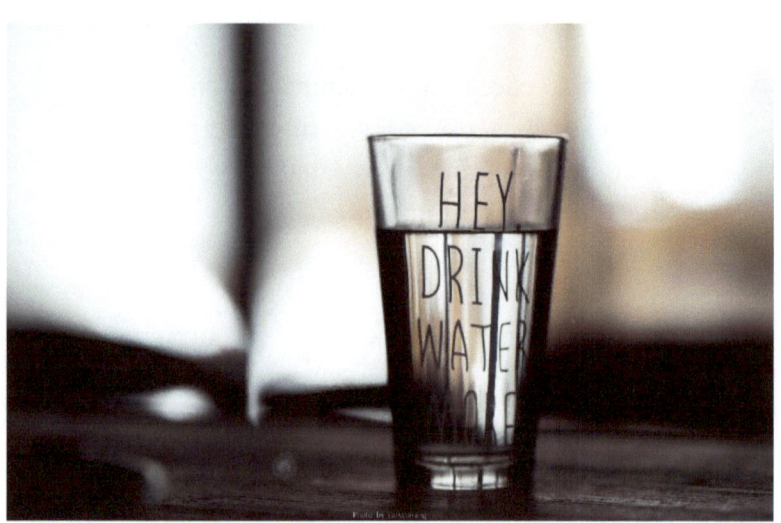

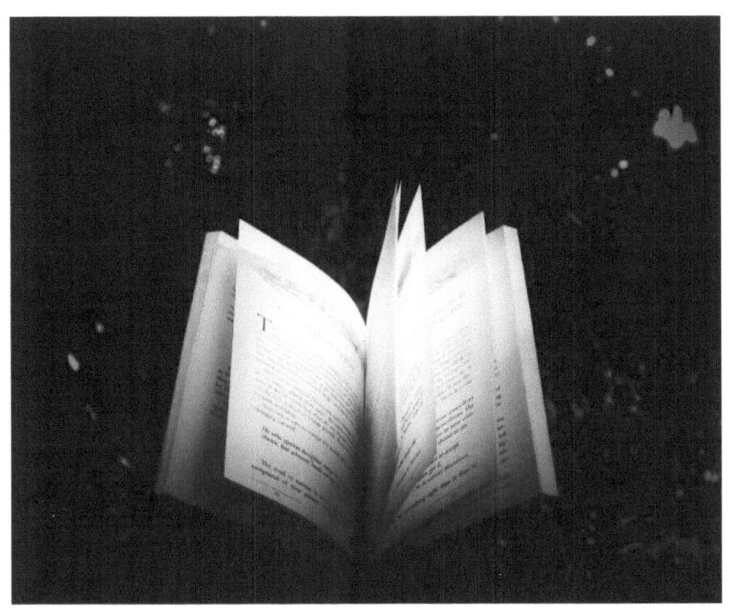

STEP 5
READ, READ, READ!

What books are you digging your nose into these days? Anything on personal development? What are the areas of study that most interest you?

One of those most forgotten but important things that we should be doing is reading. It's like most of us forget what a book is once we've graduated from school. The most successful people in the world are not only writing books but they are also reading them; that's because they understand that knowledge is wealth and applied knowledge is power.

THE BENEFITS

Reading helps to not only expand your knowledge bank, but it also widens your vocabulary. If you are looking to improve your focus, then reading should be your go to method for developing the ability to concentrate well. Reading is this neat thing we do to feed details to our mind that places images in our head, helping to improve memory.

The benefits to reading can be and are astounding, this is why including it into your daily routine can improve your life drastically.

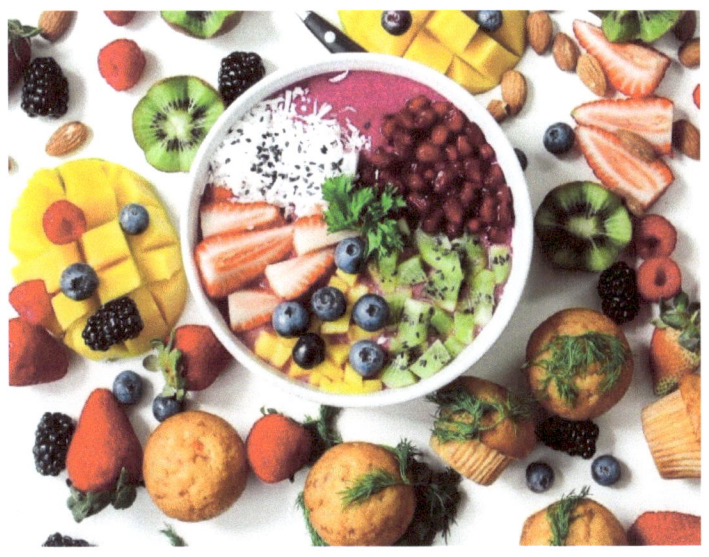

STEP 6
SHAKE UP A SMOOTHIE!

Do you enjoy the fresh taste of a delicious smoothie? If so, then this will be the best step yet!

Each day, I start my morning with an energizing, skin freshening, heart healthy smoothie to feed my mind, body and spirit.

You get out from your body what you put in. If you feed your body healthy things that are packed with nutrients and vitamins, then what you can expect is a great figure as well as beautiful skin and a body full of energy!

LOOK & FEEL BETTER NAKED

The right blends of fruit mixed with some healthy protein can increase your energy and build your stamina in order to live a better life!

Here is a list of Smoothies from Women's Health that you might want to add to your diet, which can help aide you in the areas of your skin, heart, health, eyes and can also help you shed fat Fast!

- Eye Heart Orange – made with orange juice, mango, banana, carrots and ice cubes

- The Grape Foundation – made with cashew milk, spinach, banana, frozen red grapes, almond butter and ground flaxseeds

- Oat-Nut Smoothie – made with Greek vanilla 2% yogurt, banana, almond milk, rolled oats, almond butter, honey and ice cubes

- Cranberry Almond Smoothie – made with cranberries, almond butter, unsweet cranberry juice, 2% Greek yogurt and blackberries

- Cinnamon Brain Booster – raw soaked cashews, almond or coconut milk, rolled oats, honey, ground cinnamon, ground turmeric and ice cubes

There is more where this came from… for more smoothie recipes, visit my website at www.mysacredpleasures.com.

PROTEIN

Protein makes up about 15% of a person's body weight and is essential to building muscle mass. This nutrient is composed of amino acids, which are organic compounds made up of carbon, hydrogen, nitrogen, oxygen and sulfur. Proteins are used to make not only muscles, but tendons, organs and skin.

According to the National Institute of Health, amino acids are the building blocks of muscle mass. All of that information to say that protein is vital to your diet if you want to shed some weight and build a toned-up body. The average amount of protein intake should be about 56 grams for men and 46 grams for women in a day.

When protein is broken down in the body, it helps to fuel muscle mass and increases the effectiveness of your metabolism. So, feed your body right! 😊

Have you ever heard that saying, you are what you eat? So why not be someone firm, toned, whole and fresh!

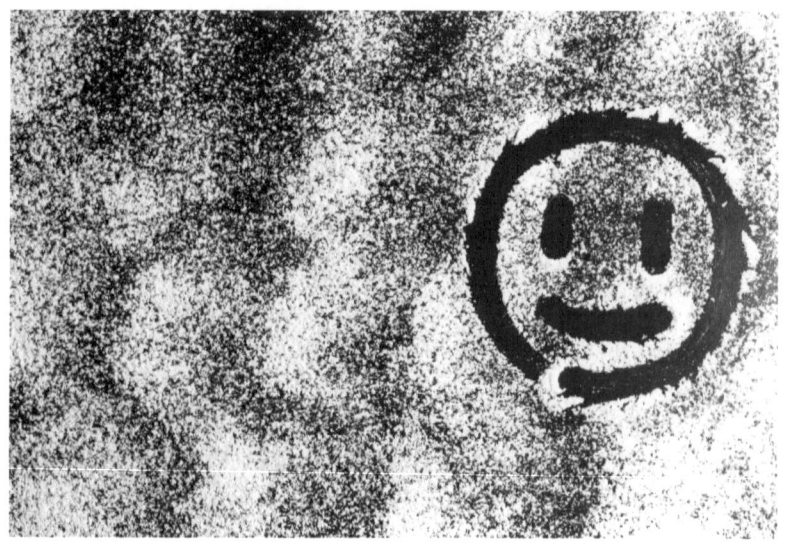

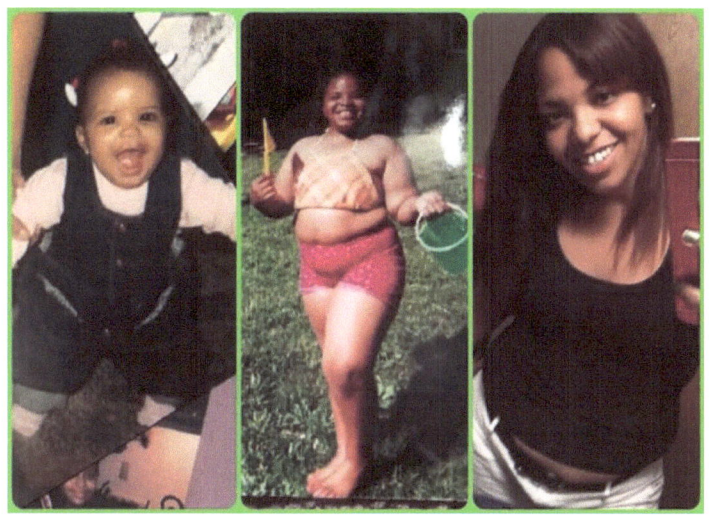

DIARY OF A FAT GIRL

MY STORY

As far back as I can remember, I've been fat. My
family likes to tell these terrible stories about how I
"liked tight" as a kid, I was even nicknamed after a
food… green-bean. Don't get me wrong, there is
nothing wrong with a little humor here and there; but
let's be honest, as an adult, tight-fitting clothes just
aren't cute anymore and neither are food names.

There was a time in my life where I tried imagining myself skinny, it was almost impossible to even picture it in my mind. At times, I would sit back and watch as the skinny girls got picked first during recess, first for dates and even won all the awards in school. At some point, I decided that enough was enough, I was no longer going to care about being fat, I'd love me just the way I was. I guess, I just decided to follow the advice that everyone around me was dishing out, *"You have to love you, Tre,"* they'd say.

This was the biggest piece of bull-crap to me at the time. How could I love me when I was no where near the happiness I was seeking? How could I love me when everyone around me was skinny and made me stick out like a sore thumb? Yes, I was sweet and friendly. Yes, everyone wanted to be my friend, but that was it. So, okay, I settled for the person in the fat suit.

Years went by and I was now satisfied with the idea of being fat. I was doomed and there was nothing that anyone could do about it. People always said things like, *"You're just big boned."* Yeah, that should have made me feel better. Honestly, how can a statement like that make me feel any better? It just made me think of myself as a T-Rex with huge bones. Why did God do this to me? Why couldn't I be thin and fit like the rest of the girls?

MY TRUTH

You see, I graduated from high school and reached 330lbs. I had given up on being fit and just let myself go. Somewhere deep within me was a person who genuinely loved life and wanted to be happy and fit, but that person seemed so far away. Because there was no easy way out of this, I gave in and grew bigger and bigger.

It wasn't until I gave birth to my child, Paije, that I decided it was truly time to find that inner me. Being overweight was a dis-ease that I could not let her see me bear. I had let everything that everyone around me was saying feed that noise in my head telling me that being in shape was impossible for me. I remember that there were even times that I'd watch 'The Biggest Loser' on tv and tell myself that I could not do it, I gave into being a loser forever.

After allowing defeat to overtake me for so long, I finally received the answer to all my problems in the biggest way possible… the realization of my testimony.

MY REVELATION

When I was finally ready shed the weight, I'd taken on meditation as a daily habit. At the time, my mind seemed like the only thing that I could control. After about 3 weeks of regular stillness, this awkward feeling came over me and it's as if the world were standing still. I remember the day like it was yesterday. I had just awoken in a new body, lighter on my feet and super energized. I jumped out of bed and threw on my work clothes, anxious to tell someone about my revelation. At the time, I wasn't really able to pinpoint the source of my energy, I just went with it.

On my way to work, everything seemed to be moving in slow motion. The traffic was flowing more smoothly and the people around me seemed to be genuinely happy that day. There was a feeling of ecstasy creeping up my back as I realized what could have been happening, an Awakening to my spirit. In that moment, it's as if the world was standing still and I was the only one here.

When I got to work, I was so excited about this new me that I was sharing with nearly anyone who would listen. Honestly, they probably thought I was crazy… but I didn't care, I had reached a place of inner peace.

FAT2FAB

Months had gone by and I'd gotten a new job, new car and a new home. Since my awakening, I'd manifested an overall better-quality life for myself. Once again, those negative perpetual thoughts about my physical appearance began to creep up again. This time, I was prepared. When those self-defeating thoughts came to attack, I was ready and armored with weights to fall into my natural state of being.

Side note: most people have no clue what I mean when I say, "natural state," and what it means is that we were perfect when we came into this physical body. We came here with a purpose and that was to learn and discover in order to lead. Anything that we Believe about ourselves is all made up by our own perception based on paradigms.

That, my friend, is exactly what happened for me. I realized the fat that was manifesting on my body was only there because I'd been hiding my true self, my true feelings and allowing the abuse, neglect and obesity to become the qualities that defined me.

As a child, as most obese children, I developed the fat suit as a way of protecting myself from the outside world. This gave me the safety net that I lacked as a kid and those sweet foods became my comfort.

I AM...

Today, I stand strong. I walk my journey with my head held high and honey, I slay! Never again will I allow the words of others to influence my decision to love me. I have managed to overcome trauma in my life in order to heal and forgive so that I could break through where I was stuck in my life.

I understand more than ever, now, the importance of loving yourself and giving the upmost attention to the things that you want more of in your life. You are your own best friend and when you recognize yourself as such, things will begin to fall into place... or fall off.

Thank you for reading My Story and I pray for strength, endurance and guidance for you as you begin your journey from #Fat2Fab.

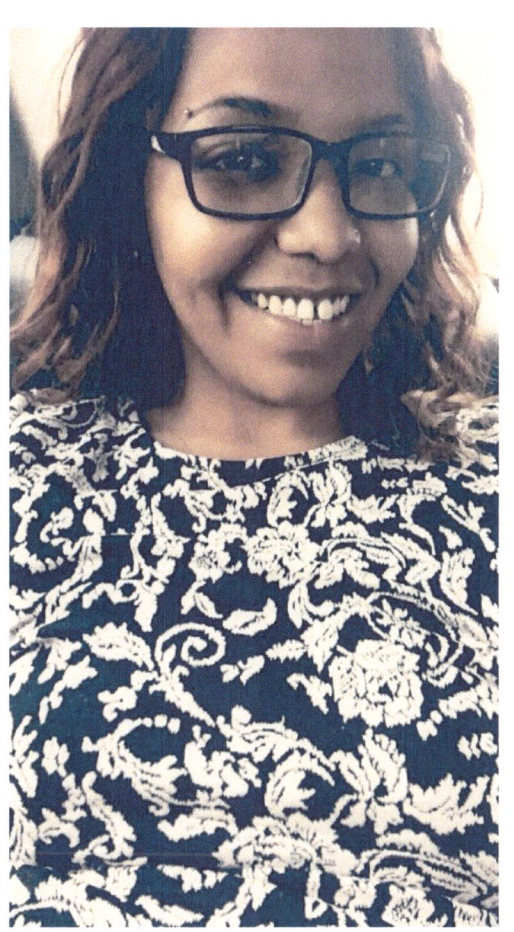